Other books by Author
(Now available on Kindle and in Paper Back)

Recipes from the Kitchens of Cosmic Pizza and Simply Delicious Pizza

Recipes from the Kitchen of The Chocolate Martini

So You Want To Open a Restaurant Expanded Addition
Includes Recipes from the Kitchens of Cosmic Pizza and Simply Delicious Pizza as well as Recipes from the Kitchen of The Chocolate Martini into this one book

So You Want To Open a Restaurant
This guide includes Spread Sheet Management Tools as well as information on lease negotiation, advertising, marketing and plating. It also includes or menu.

Live Without Stress

Kefir, Probiotics and Health Benefits of homemade Kefir

About the Author

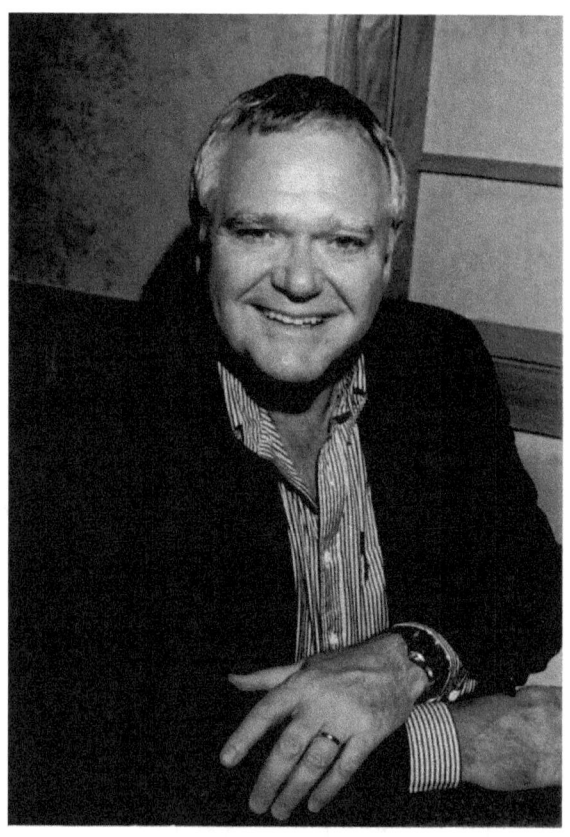

The author has owned Real Estate and Mortgage companies, 8 Restaurants, Legal Document companies, Marketing and Advertising companies, Marketing and Manufacturing companies as well as The Human Touch School of the Healing Arts and Kefir World a supplier of Kefir grains and kits for making Kefir at home.

ACKNOWLEDGEMENTS

So many people that have helped me along the way and it's time to acknowledge them!

Randal Churchill and Maureen Mulder of Hypnotherapy Institute,

Orman Mcgill, Master Hypnotherapist and author

Dr. E Bauman, Human Touch Nutritional Instructor

Mr. Sun Yi, Guang An Men Hospital, Beijing, China- Energy Work

Dr. Zang Tao, China Academy of Traditional Chinese Medicine, Guang An Men Hospital, Beijing, China- Tuina

Dr. Yan Neng-An, Guang An Men Hospital, Beijing, China- Orthapedics Dept.

Peter J, Bower, MD, Human Touch School Instructor

Usui Reiki Master Sandi Levin, 3rd in line from Reiki Master Virginia W. Samdahl

Milton Erickson, Stanislov Groff, Edgar Cayce, BHAGWAN SHREE Rajneesh, The Dali Lama

Pam Alvarez, who reintroduced me to holistic thinking

Babette Garfield McCall, who has been with me as an equal partner in life, love and education, truly none of this would have been possible without her by my side pointing the way.

Lastly the GENERATIONS of Kefir makers who have continued to make and teach others the wonders of Kefir making at home and the researchers and scientists who have proven how probiotics can give you a healthier life! Homemade Kefir has more probiotics than any other product available in stores today at a fraction of their cost, be they pill, capsule or drink!

Introduction

I started making Kefir after my wife and I had used some probiotic capsules and saw and felt dramatic changes in our physical selves. Both internally and externally.

First, let me tell you a little about ourselves and our health as it will help you understand our feelings about Kefir and why we started supplying Kefir making kits for home use.

At this writing I'm 68, a Vietnam Veteran with a service related disability currently rated at 50%. I have Knee and Back damage as well as feeling loss from nerve damage in my legs and feet. Some days are more challenging than others and I keep a collection of canes at home and in my car for when they're needed and have medication for inflammation, pain and cramping.

Now let me tell you about my wife. She's 3 years younger than me and a 14 year survivor of Breast Cancer, who after her operation chose not to do chemo or radiation. Like many her age she has a couple of pills to take on a daily basis.

She was feeling a bit sluggish. Given her history we pay attention as to how we feel. She just wasn't present.

Needless to say we really don't like taking pills and started looking into probiotics after our local cable company showed an advertisement about a probiotic product. In a sense it was more of an infomercial since it told us how, unlike our ancestors, we are eating much more processed foods and now have the wrong types of bacteria in our gut, digestive tract.

We have 80% bad and 20% good which is the exact opposite of what we should have. That this bad bacteria causes inflammation, sluggishness, heart disease, yeast infections and many, many more physical problems in all ages.

We tried some probiotics capsules and both of us had an instant improvement. The drug store capsules were expensive and contained about 10 friendly bacteria totaling about 30 billion. Most never make it to the intestines because of stomach acid.

I started researching probiotics and how they were made. Mostly because of how much the capsules cost so if I could make them at home I wanted to try. I can't help myself, it's who I am.

That's how I discovered homemade Kefir. It's easy to make, low cost and contains at least 5 times more probiotics than any capsule. With something like a trillion per glass. (Beats 30 billion by miles!)

While I'm going to give you the History, Myth and Folk lore, and a great deal of scientific research information my main goal is to give you the information to make Kefir at home. We do offer Kefir starter and instructions on our website, www.kefirworld.com .

You must obtain starter Kefir Grains to make Kefir.

Let me describe Kefir. Kefir looks like lumpy plain Yogurt. Some people say the lumps look like small bit of Cauliflower or Cottage Cheese. They call this Kefir Grains

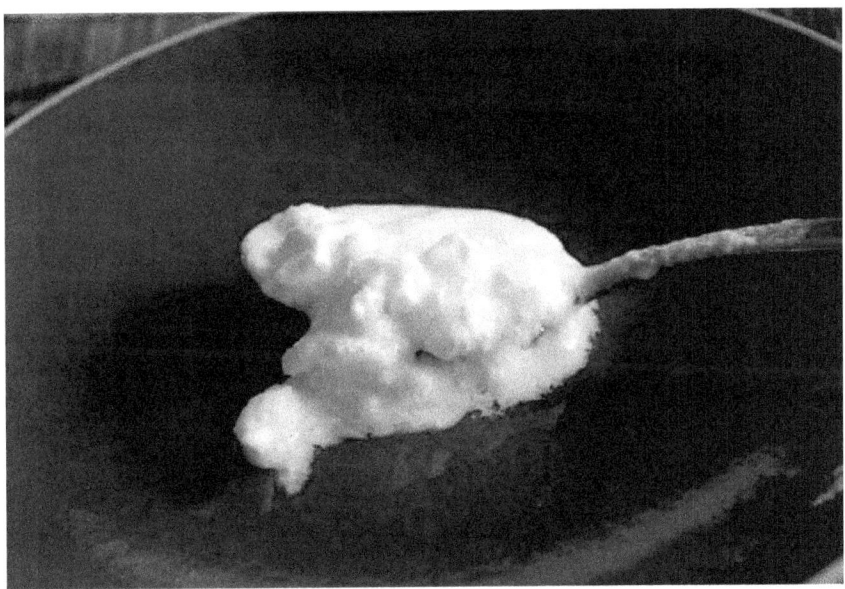

It's a fermentation process, and the grains are filtered out and reused over and over again. The strained liquid is the Kefir you drink and many people use it in smoothie like drinks or with flavored creams. I drink it plain but Babette likes Hazelnut cream added.

Historical Research

When you search the internet and get website after website saying almost the same thing, then there has to be an original source. While I think I found one or two in Russian websites, where Kefir originated, I can't be sure but I'm close.

On some of the following pages you will see research references from Doctors, Researchers, Scientists, and Clinics. Any research referenced will have additional proofs in the back pages of this book.

There are a number of health related claims made about Kefir and while I can make anecdotal statements about what Babette and I have experienced, were are not Doctors.

Our feelings for a healthy life style and alternative medicine goes back to the 1980s when we first met.

I had recently left the high stressed world of business and Babette had just sold her interest in a wholesale fish poultry business that had an oyster bar and restaurant as a part of it.

Needless to say our thoughts melded together and we bought a school.

The Human Touch School of the Healing Arts

The Human Touch was our Post-Secondary Education School in California. We taught massage, hypnosis and nutrition. Our staff included a MD, a DO, a PhD and others with a vast knowledge in their areas of expertise.

Our student body was made up of Doctors and Nurses who were required to earn continuing education credits as well as others who wished to open practices.

Some of the instructors, at my request and through a grant from our school, studied in China at the China Academy of Traditional Chinese Medicine, Guang An Men Hospital, Beijing, China.

Doctors in China had to be in practice for 12 years to attend this teaching hospital.

My wife and I along with one other instructor from our school studied there. Later some of the Chinese Doctors came to our school as visiting Instructors.

One of the only things I had trouble accepting about our studies in China was how some treatments would be effective for so many unrelated problems. A silly example would be your head hurts and you have the hiccups. Push this acupressure point and both go away.

So when I read that probiotics, Kefir, is helpful for inflammation, ulcers, yeast infections, helps prevents heart attacks and a host of other diseases, well you get what I mean.. Hence the extensive research.

I'm happy to say that the research does bear out that probiotics do what has been written about them in some remarkable ways.

As an example, 80% of your immune system's ability to fight harmful bacteria is located, you guested it, in your gut. The name "Probiotics" mean Pro Life. "Antibiotics" is Against Life. That's why we're told to take probiotics after we've had an antibiotic. The good fauna has been killed along with the bad fauna. We need to restore the "GOOD".

Homemade Kefir is a wonderful way to do so and is superior to any store bought processed kefir product and much less expensive and has a larger group of good strains of bacteria, (37 from homemade verses maybe 10 in processed kefir and only 3 to 10 in Capsules).

Having owned a school that taught nutrition courses helped us see the value of homemade Kefir, once we discovered it. We hope that this informational book will lead you to a wonderful and healthy way to put natural probiotics into your life.

When you're finished reading you'll know where to get Kefir and how to make it at home, Promise!

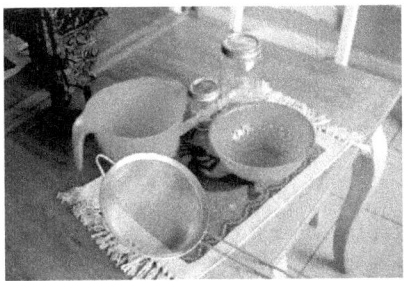

All the things you need to make Kefir at home. I use the stainless steel strainer to get a smoother drink. My wife doesn't like the little Kefir Grains in her Kefir.

Above all This book is presented to help you have a heathier life.

Making Kefir is very very simple using everyday milk. We use organic milk.

TABLE OF CONTENTS

History of Kefir

Kefir (кефир) is a drink made of fermented milk not unlike yogurt, whose origins lie with nomadic shepherds living on the slopes of the North Caucasus Mountains. Today, kefir is the most popular fermented milk in Russia. Late in the 20th century, (1988) , kefir accounted for between 65% and 80% of total fermented milk sales in Russia, that's over 1.2 million tons of Kefir!

Kefir's popularity has spread from Eastern Europe and is now regularly consumed in North America, Europe, Australia, and the United Kingdom. This kefir is <u>pasteurized</u> after fermentation and can be found in many stores and supermarkets. It's also being produced on a large scale in countries that once made up the Soviet Union or block, as well as Czechoslovakia, Hungary, Poland, Finland, Norway, Sweden, Switzerland, Germany, and even as far away as Southeast Asia.

Kefir has also been enjoyed in Chile for over a century, likely brought to South America by waves of immigrants from Eastern Europe or the former Ottoman Empire. Flavored varieties have been developed and are especially popular in the United States.

Kefir: Myths and Folklore

Some scholars believe that kefir grains were in fact the "manna" described in the Bible as being provided by God to feed the Israelites as they wandered the desert for forty years before Moses led them to the Promised Land.

Some scholars also think that kefir is what angels taught Abraham to make, which he credited for his long life and many children.

The more common legend among the Islamic people living on the northern slopes of the Caucasus Mountains is that Mohammed gave kefir grains to Orthodox Christians, thereby teaching them to make kefir.

They called Kefir grains, the "Grains of the Prophet."

Kefirs name may have come from the Turkish word "keyif" which means "good feeling" because traditionally, drinking kefir was associated with general well-being and long life.

Kefir grains were jealously guarded by their owners. They believed the grains would lose their potency if the secret of their use became known.

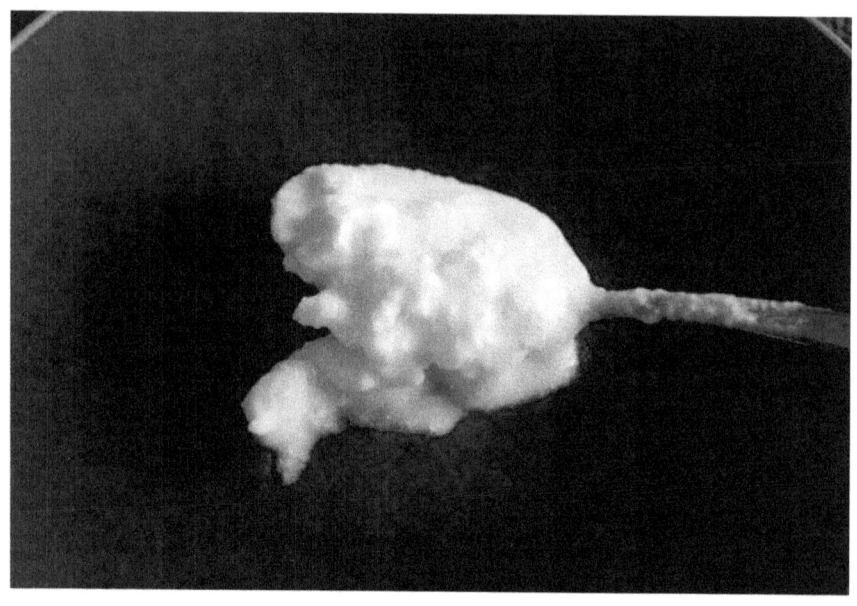

Kefir Grains

Thus, Kefir grains were secretly passed from one generation to the next, closely guarded as part of the wealth of each family within the tribe, and although foreigners were sometimes given kefir to drink, Marco Polo recounts tasting kefir in the book of his eastern travels, the method of making kefir was kept secret and the drink was all but forgotten, until the 19th century.

It cannot be overlooked that kefir grains really can be described as "magical".

Despite intensive research spanning well over a century and many attempts to produce kefir grains from pure or mixed cultures normally found in the grains, no successful results have been reported to this day, likely because so very little is known about the way in which the kefir grains form.

When I look at Kefir Grains I see a structure similar to what we call in the U.S "Cottage Cheese". The grains even taste a bit like cheese when you chew one.

Originally How Kefir was Made

The most ancient methods of making kefir were far from complicated. Fresh milk from cows, goats, or sheep was poured into bags made of goat or sheepskin. Now add the Kefir Grains or kefir culture to the bag. It was then suspended in the door way and sun during the day. When the sun went down, the bag was brought inside and hung near the door. Each person passing in or out of the doorway would be expected to push or squeeze the bag, thus helping ensure that the milk and kefir grains remained well mixed as the milk fermented.

As kefir was consumed, more milk was added to the bag so that the process could continue uninterrupted as it had for over a thousand years. This process has descended through the ages from kefir grains first used many generations ago.

Occasionally, kefir was made in clay pots, wooden buckets, or even vats of oak, but the most traditional method of making kefir was in goat or sheep skin bags.

Shepherds would make their own kefir as they traveled. When leaving home, they would take skins of kefir with them on their treks across the slopes, adding fresh milk from the animals they herded to replace what they consumed. As the shepherd moved, the milk would mix with the kefir grains and ferment into the mildly self-carbonated beverage that they drank and simultaneously used to make more kefir.

Word of Kefir spreads

During the Victorian Age, news spread that the use of kefir was successful in the treatment of such varied diseases as tuberculosis, intestinal and stomach diseases.

Russian doctors began studying kefir's properties in earnest. Although the first studies on the benefits of kefir were published at the end of the 19th century, kefir was still very difficult to find as, without the kefir grains, Kefir was impossible to make. Demand for Kefir had grown!

Members of the "All Russian Physician's Society" were determined to obtain the elusive kefir grains in order to make kefir for their patients on an industrial scale and approached the Blandov brothers who owned and ran the largest Moscow Dairy and also owned cheese-manufacturing factories in the town of Kislovodsk in the

Northern Caucasus region where Kefir was found. They wanted them to procure kefir grains for the project.

What happened next is a story straight out of a romance novel or an adventure film.

One of the brothers, Nikolai, sent an employee,

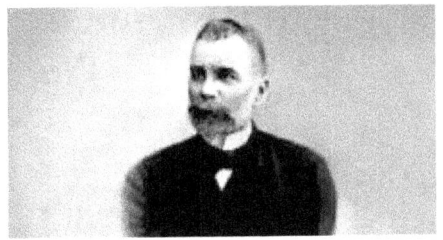 Nikolai Balandov

Irina Sakharova, who was beautiful, young and willing to go to the court of Prince Bek-Mirza Barchorov, the local Prince, with instructions to charm him and obtain some kefir grains.

While the Prince greatly desired Irina, he feared violating religious folklore laws and refused to give away the "Grains of the Prophet" even to her.

Recognizing that her mission was a failure, Irina and the men accompanying her left to return to Kislovodsk. The Prince, however, was not going to let Irina escape; and as it was a local custom to steal a bride prior to marrying her, The Prince sent men from a local mountain tribe to capture her.

Following her kidnapping, Irina remained silent and would not address the Princes proposal of marriage, which gave her employers enough time to organize a daring mission to save her from the Prince.

After Irina's rescue, Prince Bek-Mirza Barchorov was brought before Tsar Nicholas II who ruled Russia.

The Prince was ordered to give Irina compensation for the kidnapping and other insults that she was forced to endure, the Prince gave Irina ten pounds of kefir grains.

Following the royal ruling, the priceless kefir grains were taken to the Moscow Dairy owned by the Blandov brothers and the first bottles of kefir ever manufactured commercially were offered for sale in Moscow in September 1908.

However, it wasn't until the 1930s that the manufacture of kefir began on a large scale.

The first kefir-making process wasn't without its complications. The first commercial product was made by growing a quantity of kefir grains in milk and then straining them out before allowing the cultured milk to ferment larger batches of fresh milk.

Unfortunately, the finished product was greatly inferior to traditionally produced kefir. They then went back to making smaller batches the traditional way.

It wasn't until the 1950s that the commercial process was perfected. The employees of the "All-Union Dairy Research Institute" (VNIMI) developed a better method which included stirring the mix of kefir grains and milk in a large vessel and permitting the entire process, consisting of fermentation, coagulation, agitation of the mixture, ripening of the kefir, and its resting to take place in the same container prior to being bottled and sold.

In 1973, when Irina Sakharova was 85 years old, the Minister of Food and Industry of the Soviet Union sent her a letter acknowledging her part and thanking her for bringing kefir to the Russian people.

Though it is believed that kefir originated in the Caucasus Mountains, similar lactic acid fermented milk beverages are also cultivated elsewhere in the world.

Other traditional fermented milk beverages are made in Taiwan, northern Europe, central Asia and Africa.

In all cases the beverage has enhanced the health of those who have taken them. Only Kefir has had the extensive medical and scientific research proving the health benefits.

Health Benefits of Kefir

The people of the Caucasus region are famed for their extraordinary longevity and many accredit this to their regular consumption of kefir.

In fact, in the early 1970s, National Geographic magazine wanted a specialist to visit, study, and write an article about the long and healthy lives of the region that Kefir was found in.

They asked Dr. Leaf, a Professor of Clinical Medicine at Harvard University and Chief of Medical Services at Massachusetts General Hospital to do it.

His goal was to locate and study those societies where a large percentage of elder citizens retained their faculties, were vigorous, and enjoyed their lives.

His goal was to understand the key factors that influence human prospects for long and healthy life. What they ate, their life style.

Dr. Leaf journeys were later made into a series of articles that appeared in National Geographic magazine beginning in 1973.

One of the regions in the series was the Caucasus mountains, specifically a place known as Abkhasia, in what was then the Soviet Union.

Prior to Dr Leafs journey to the region Life magazine had run an article with photos of Shirali Muslimov, said to be 161 years old. In one of the photos, Muslimov was shown with his third wife. He told the reporter that he had married her when he was 110.

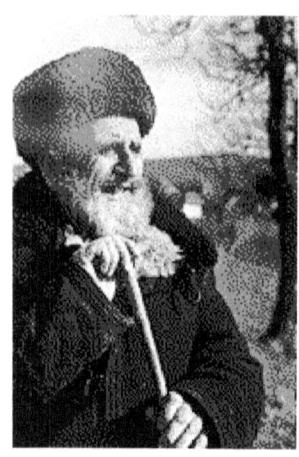 Shirali Muslimov

Dr. Leaf said "We were eager to see the centenarians and Abkhasia seemed to be the place to go."

Dr. Leaf studied the people of Abkhasia and wrote, "Certainly no area in the world has the reputation for long-lived people to match that of the Caucasus in southern Russia."

A 1970 census had established Abkhasia, then an autonomous region within Soviet Georgia, as the longevity capital of the world and it is found between the Black Sea and the main Caucasus range, with Russia on the north and Georgia to the south.

The Soviet press announced that Shirali Muslimov was 168 years old, and the government commemorated the assertion by putting his face on a postage stamp.

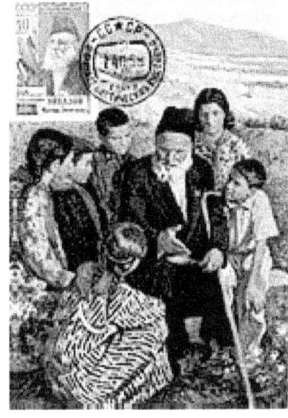

Hospitals in the former USSR used kefir to treat conditions ranging from atherosclerosis, allergic disease, metabolic and digestive disorders, tuberculosis, cancer, and gastrointestinal disorders.

Modern Day Facts

Recently there was an article in the "HOW TO HANDBOOK health section of a Martha Stewart magazine, Go With Your Gut". It talks about how emerging research on Probiotic bacteria which lives in our stomach or digestive system and how the flora keeps us healthy and feeling well.

In the article Dr. Liponis, the medical director of Canyon Ranch health resorts states that new data shows that the probiotics in our digestive system is critical to our well-being, our general wellness. That our digestive tract is home to 80% of our immune cells, 80%! He said that when it's necessary to take antibiotics remember that anti biotics kills all flora, healthy and bad and that because of the killing of good flora there is a chance for complications like yeast infection, skin rash and allergic reaction.

Always use probiotics to repopulate the healthy flora. Over the counter probiotic supplements are helpful, they usually contain 2 to 10 good strains of bacteria within the 30 billion per dose capsules. However what you want is to ingest real live food like Kefir with its 37 plus strains of good flora and 1 trillion live probiotics flora whenever you can.

Dr. A Junger, a New York Cardiologist and author of Clean Gut (Harper, 2013) states that when our gut is efficiently functioning, in balance with good flora, we feel so much better.

Our digestive system has about 100 Trillion bacteria, sometimes called "Flora". This flora out numbers human cells 10 to 1!

There's good and bad bacteria, flora each excreting compounds into our system which can have a positive or negative effect on our health stated Dr. Hazen, the Chair of Cellular and Molecular Medicine at the Cleveland Clinic.

It was also stated by Ph.D. Proctor of the Human Microbiome Project at the National Institute of Health that to have a healthy gut you should avoid eating foods high in sugar, fats, and processed foods which cause gas, discomfort, bloating and Inflammation.

Bad flora allows Non-nutritive materials to slip into our bodies and effect how we feel. Good bacteria aid in the digestion, our well-being and general good health and helps nutrients and healthy compounds get into the blood stream.

Studies of twins, published in Nature, found that it is possible that bad bacteria can cause obesity. When gut bacteria from obese twins were introduced to mice they turned fat. When gut bacteria was introduced from thin twins the mice stayed thin.

The study also suggested that the obese and diabetic patients lacked diversity of bacteria, not enough good bacterial strains.

The Cleveland Clinic found that some bad bacteria, when digesting eggs and meat, can make a compound that aids the clogging of arteries. Dr. Hazen stated that this is why some unhealthy eaters get heart disease and others don't.

The good news is that we can replace, swap, the bad bacteria with good bacteria within a matter of days or weeks, depending how off balance our gut flora is.

Ph.D Huang, a Metabolic Biologist at the University of California, Berkeley stated that by cultivating healthful flora, the desirable flora will kill off the bad.

Dr. Nicholas Perricone, the anti-aging skin expert who has an expensive skin care line, has called kefir a superfood because of all the good things it does.

Modern Research

In recent years, scientific studies have proven that kefir is able to stimulate the immune system, enhance lactose digestion, as well as inhibit tumors, fungi and pathogens— including the bacteria that cause most ulcers, Helicobacter pylori.

Kefir contains large numbers of probiotics, the microbes that live in our bodies and provide us with important health benefits such as boosting immunity, calming inflammation, assisting in digestion, creating amino acids and vitamins, and aiding in digestion.

Kefir, which can be made from any type of mammalian milk, also contains partially digested proteins, enzymes (including lactase, which is good for people who are lactose intolerant), vitamins (A, B1, B3, B9/folate, B12, D and vitamin K), minerals and essential amino acids.

The kefir beverage is fermented from fresh milk (can be cow, goat, ewe, buffalo, horse or even human milk) by the microorganisms contained in the living kefir grains. There have been reports that successful kefir has been made from soy milk and coconut milk, as well. Probiotics enter the kefir as part of the fermentation, but have a different microbiological mix than the grains themselves.

During fermentation, several components are produced including minute quantities of alcohol, lactic acid, carbon dioxide, enzymes and vitamins. Lactose that was originally in the milk is reduced, so many people who are lactose intolerant can drink it.

Kefir has been used for the treatment of atherosclerosis, allergies, diseases like eczema that are related to allergies, gastrointestinal disorders, tuberculosis and cancer.

As interest in probiotics has increased, the Western world has started to take an interest in finding out if there is any truth to the wide-ranging claims about kefir.

Western and Asian researchers have undertaken multiple studies with extremely encouraging results.

Immune System. Several studies have confirmed that the immune system response is enhanced by kefir, although it is not yet clear whether it is the bacteria in the kefir, metabolites produced during fermentation or an element of the kefir grains themselves that cause this effect.

A stimulated immune system is better at identifying and combatting disease. Kefir is very effective at maintaining a balanced and healthy gut microbiome, which boosts the ability of the gut to fend of pathogenic microbes.

Gastrointestinal Disturbances. Kefir consumption has been shown to be helpful both in preventing constipation as well as preventing and treating diarrhea. It has also been shown to reduce flatulence. Lactose intolerant subjects have been shown to be able to tolerate kefir without symptoms.

Allergies. It has been shown that consuming kefir has reduces asthma symptoms in mice. It can decrease the allergy response to symptom triggering allergens, according to research. Kefir has also been shown to reduce food allergies in study participants.

Anti-Inflammatory Effects. In studies on mice, kefir has been shown to reduce inflammation.

Cancer. There have been many promising studies on the effect of kefir (including the probiotics in kefir) and cancer.

The probiotics in kefir have been shown to bind to mutagens that are potentially cancer causing, thereby reducing their potential harm to the body, anti-mutagenic effects.

Those people who drink kefir regularly are statistically much less likely to get colon cancer than those who do not. It has been shown to have anti-mutagenic effects with respect to colon cancer and thus may play a role in colon cancer prevention. The kefir grains themselves have been shown to have tumor inhibiting capabilities for sarcomas, melanomas, lung and breast cancer cells, anti-carcinogenic effects. It will be really exciting to see the results from studies on cancer and probiotics that are currently underway.

Antibacterial and Antifungal. Kefir has shown anti-microbial activity against a wide range of harmful bacteria and fungi. Kefir can help to control rotavirus and Clostridium difficile (C. difficile) infections as well as ulcers related to Helicobacter pylori. It can be used as antibiotic therapy. It has been used effectively to treat travelers' diarrhea.

Research References for the above sections

Leaf, Alexander (January 1973). "Search for the Oldest People". *National Geographic*. pp. 93–118.

Farnsworth, Edward 2006, *Kefir –a Complex Probiotic*, Food Science and Technology Bulletin: Functional Foods, vol. 2, pp 1-18

Lee MY, Ahn KS, Kwon OK, Kim MJ, Kim MK, Lee IY, Oh SR, Lee HK 2007, *Anti-inflammatory and anti-allergic effect of kefir in a mouse asthma model*, **Immunobiology**, Issue 212, pp. 647–654

Hong W S, Chen Y P and Chen M J, 2010, *The Antiallergenic effect of Kefir Lactobacilli*, **Journal of Food Science**, vol. 75, no. 8, pp. 244-253

Murch, S. H. 2001. *Toll of allergy reduced by probiotics*, **Lancet** issue 357, pp 1057–59

Brady, L. J., D. D. Gallagher, and F. F. Busta. 2000. *The role of probiotic cultures in the prevention of colon cancer*. **Journal of Nutrition** vol. 130, pp 410–14

Wollowski, I., G. Rechkemmer, G., and B. L. Pool-Zobel. 2001. *Protective role of probiotics and prebiotics in colon cancer.* **American Journal of Clinical Nutrition**, vol 73(2 suppl) pp. 4515–55

kefir. dictionary.reference.com

Prescott; Harley; Klein. *Microbiology* (7th ed.). London: McGraw-Hill. p. 1040. ISBN 9780071102315.

"Wiktionary, the free dictionary: Kefir".

"Origin of KEFIR". Merriam-Webster Dictionary Online.

"kefir – Memidex dictionary/thesaurus".

"CODEX Standard for Fermented Milks #243-2003". FAO/WHO.

Handbook of Fermented Functional foods. 2nd Ed. Edward R. Farnsworth, Editor. CRC Press, 2008.

Farnworth, Edward R. (2005). "Kefir – a complex probiotic". *Food Science & Technology Bulletin: Functional Foods* **2** (1): 1–17. doi:10.1616/1476-2137.13938.

Kowsikowski, F. and Mistry, V. (1997). Cheese and Fermented Milk Foods, 3rd ed, vol. I. F. V. Kowsikowski, Westport, Conn., ISBN 0965645606.

Motegi et al.; Mazaheri, M.; Moazami, N.; Farkhondeh, A.; Fooladi, M.H.; Goltapeh, E.M. (1997). "Kefir production in Iran". *World Journal of Microbiology & Biotechnology* **13** (5): 579–581. doi:10.1023/A:1018577728412.

"Fabrication of kefir". Retrieved 12 November 2013.

"Journal of Dairy Research". Retrieved 15 November 2013.

"Journal of Dairy Research". *Journal of Dairy Research* **68** (4): 639–652. November 2001.

Sedova NN; Sedova NN (1974). "Detection and quantitive determination of Shigella sonnei in milk and milk products.". *Voprosy Pitaniya* **4**: 42–45.

Kneifel, W; Mayer, HK (1991). "Vitamin profiles of kefirs made from milks of different species". *International Journal of Food Science & Technology* **26** (4): 423–428. doi:10.1111/j.1365-2621.1991.tb01985.x.

Hertzler, Steven R.; Clancy, Shannon M. (May 2003). "Kefir improves lactose digestion and tolerance in adults with lactose maldigestion". *J Am Diet Assoc* (Elsevier, Inc.) **103** (5): 582–587. doi:10.1053/jada.2003.50111. PMID 12728216. Retrieved 2007-06-10.

"Kefir may bolster lactose tolerance in intolerant people". *ScienceDaily*. 2003-05-30. Retrieved 2010-06-05.

Maeda, H; Zhu, X; Omura, K; Suzuki, S; Kitamura, S (2004-12-30). "Effects of an exopolysaccharide (kefiran) on lipids, blood pressure, blood glucose, and constipation". *BioFactors* (IOS Press) **22** (1–4): 197–200. doi:10.1002/biof.5520220141. PMID 15630283. Retrieved 2007-06-10.

Liu, Je-Ruei; Chen, Ming-Ju; Lin, Chin-Win (2005). "Antimutagenic and antioxidant properties of milk-kefir and soymilk-kefir". *J Agric Food Chem* **53** (7): 2467–2474. doi:10.1021/jf048934k. PMID 15796581.

Maeda, H; Zhu, X; Suzuki, S; Suzuki, K; Kitamura, S (2004-08-25). "Structural characterization and biological activities of an exopolysaccharide kefiran produced by Lactobacillus kefiranofaciens

WT-2B(T)". *Journal of Agricultural and Food Chemistry* (American Chemical Society) **52** (17): 5533–8. doi:10.1021/jf049617g. PMID 15315396. Retrieved 2007-06-10.

Abraham, Analía G.; de Antoni, Graciela L. (May 1999). "Characterization of kefir grains grown in cows' milk and in soy milk". *Journal of Dairy Research* (Cambridge University Press) **66** (2): 327–333. doi:10.1017/S0022029999003490. PMID 10376251. Retrieved 2007-06-09.

Chen, T.-H.; Chen, M.-J.; Chen, K.-N.; Liu, J.-R.; Chen, M.-J. (2009). "Microbiological and chemical properties of kefir manufactured by entrapped microorganisms isolated from kefir grains". *Journal of Dairy Science* **92** (7): 3002–3013. doi:10.3168/jds.2008-1669. PMID 19528577.

Motaghi, M.; Mazaheri, M.; Moazami, N.; Farkhondeh, A.; Fooladi, M. H.; Goltapeh, E. M. (1997). "Short Communication: Kefir production in Iran". *World Journal of Microbiology & Biotechnology* **13** (5): 579–581. doi:10.1023/A:1018577728412.

Marshall VM, Cole WM, Brooker BE (1984). "Observations on the structure of kefir grains and the distribution of the microflora". *J Appl Bacteriol* **57** (3): 491–7. doi:10.1111/j.1365-2672.1984.tb01415.x.

Sheng-Yao Wang and Kun-Nan Chen and Yung-Ming Lo and Ming-Lun Chiang and Hsi-Chia Chen and Je-Ruei Liu and Ming-Ju Chen (2012). "Investigation of microorganisms involved in biosynthesis of the kefir grain". *Food Microbiology* **32** (2): 274–285. doi:10.1016/j.fm.2012.07.001.

Katz, Sandor Ellix (2003). *Wild Fermentation: The Flavor, Nutrition, and Craft of Live-Culture Foods*. Chelsea Green Publishing Company. ISBN 1-931498-23-7.

Margulis, Lynn. *Sex, Death and Kefir*; August 1994; Scientific American Magazine, p. 96.

Fermented Foods: Kefir, from the National Center for Home Food Preservation

"Kephir". *Collier's New Encyclopedia*. 1921.

"Kephir". *New International Encyclopedia*. 1905.

Kefir making sequence

Equipment needs (see pictures below)

- A plastic or stainless steel strainer
- A stainless steel pan, Glass or plastic bowl large enough to hold the amount of Kefir being strained after the 18 hour first fermentation.
- 1 quart sized Ball Jar, (remember there are 2 quarts to a half gallon of milk).
- Kefir Grain Starter, Our Kefir Starter is from organic raw cow's milk from an organic farm.
- Milk, (any type of ORGANIC milk can be used, or raw milk from Cows, Sheep or Goat, if you can find it. Homogenized whole organic milk is also great. Even 2% Organic milk Homogenized and Ultra Pasteurized makes a wonderful Kefir.

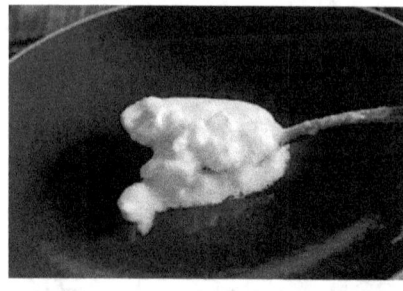

Kefir Grains

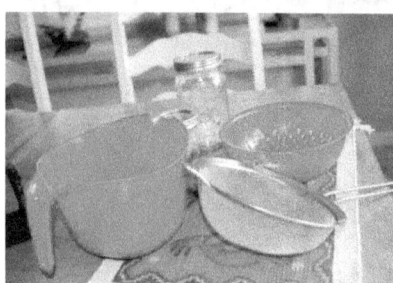

Strainers

Let's get started

Your Kefir Starter grains comes to you by mail in a flexible container filled with air and enough organic milk to feed it while it was in transit to you.

When it arrives, simply place it in your refrigerator, (Kefir should never be frozen), until you are ready to fill jars and start the first fermentation cycle of 18 hours. (If storing, add a small amount of fresh milk to feed it first!)

So, as an example, if you start to fill you Quart jars at 6pm. this evening, the first fermentation cycle of 18 hours will end at 12 noon tomorrow.

The second fermentation cycle is 6 hours, so it ends at 6pm. In other words, 24 hours from when you started.

1- First fermentation

- Remove Kefir Starter from refrigerator and divide Kefir Grains and liquid, (the Kefir Grains look like small pieces of Cauliflower or Cottage cheese), equally into the Quart (32 oz.) Jars you will be using to make your Kefir.
- You don't need a lot of Kefir Grains per jar so feel free to make from 2 to 4 quarts from this starter.

- Add milk to make jars ¾ full. Then, slowly screw the jar tops down until you feel resistance, then ease off so that the top is still loose. It should easily move when lifted but not come off.
- Place in a dark area or cover with thick towel on counter where it will not be moved. The temperature range should be between 75 to 85 degrees.

After 18 hours of fermentation in a dark area or under cover, seal jar tight and shake up to release any kefir grains on bottom. Then strain to remove Kefir Grains.

2. Straining

There are a lot of people who feel only plastic strainers should be used. With the development of modern stainless steel, that is no longer true. Feel comfortable using either.

- Place strainer over Stainless Steel, Glass or Plastic bowl and slowly pour Kefir from jars. Depending on the size of the strainer holes you may need to shake the strainer a bit.
- Remove Kefir Grains from strainer and place in the 32oz. Kefir Starter jar with a little of the kefir that was just made and fresh milk until ¾ full for storage of the Kefir grains needed for your next cycle. Store them in a Quart jar with top sealed tight for up to 10 days.

- When kefir grains are washed with clean, cold water and dried on cloth or paper for 2 days at room temperature, they can then be stored in a dry, cool place for well over a year and still stay active. They can also be freeze-dried.

If you are making more Kefir right away, then place equal amounts of Kefir Grains in new jars with some of the strained Kefir and cover grains with fresh milk so jar are ¾ filled.

- Place the lids on loosely as before and return the newly made Kefir Grain back in the dark area or under the dark towel and repeat 18 hour first fermentation cycle.

3. The second Fermentation Cycle, 6 hours

- Now pour the strained Kefir that just completed its 18 hour first fermentation cycle back into the jars it came out of.

- Wipe the top of the jar and screw on tops TIGHTLY. Place back in dark area or under a towel as before.
- Mark the jars with the number 2 or a message that these jars are in their second fermentation and the time they will be ready.

When the 2nd fermentation cycle is over simply shake, pour some into a glass for your first taste or place in refrigerator until you're ready to have some. ENJOY!

A personal note

I started with 1 Jar and then made 3 additional jars, for a total of 4 jars which is enough for my household. The forth jar is where I store my Kefir Grains, sealed tight and in the refrigerator between making Kefir. My refrigerator is at 39 degrees and slows down the fermentation so I can store starter for 14 days. Sometimes when I have to be some place I skip the second 6 hour fermentation cycle and simply place the Kefir in my refrigerator. Because the cold slows down fermentation I wait until the next day to use that batch of Kefir.

While many websites like to sound precise and scientific, nomads were making Kefir in animal skin bags for centuries. Doing it the way I instruct allows for a consistent and wonderful product.

Long term storage is also simple. Take a spoonful of Kefir Grains and place in strainer. Run spring water, (tap water that's filtered is ok but not Chlorinated), over grains until 95 % of the milk is removed. Now place the grains and spread them on parchment paper or a cleaned and ironed cotton cloth. Cover to prevent dust from settling on grains and place aside to allow the grains to dry for 3 days. The grains will *turn a yellowish color. Now place the dried grains in a small glass container or jar and refrigerate. The grains can stay store for up to 12 months.*

To rehydrate the grains, pour milk into the storage jar, with a loose lid and place in a dark place as if you were making Kefir.

Next day change the milk, pour it off the Kefir grains. Do the same each day for 3 days and then on the fourth simply make your Kefir as normal.

How To Buy Our Kefir Kit

Kefir World offers Kefir making Starter on it's website- www.kefirworld.com.

Additionally you will find recipes for foods using kefir as well as skin care and more!

The "First Taste"

If this is your first taste of Kefir you will find it tastes a bit like plain yogurt and any small solids a bit like cheese.

Start with a small amount in your glass.

Remember you are replacing "Bad Bacteria" with "GOOD PROBIOTIC BACTERIA" and there may be a bit of gas in the beginning.

Let your body slowly get use to the "GOOD". (The gut takes a few days to replace the bad with the good).

Drink only cocktail size glasses of kefir in the beginning, at breakfast.

My wife prefers to have hers with just a touch of Hazelnut, Italian Cream or Vanilla Coffee Mate.

I usually drink it plain but sometimes I'll add some Italian Cream as well.

The Kefir is wonderful in Smoothies and I especially like kefir as a substitute for milk with berries and fruits.

www.ingramcontent.com/pod-product-compliance
Lightning Source LLC
Chambersburg PA
CBHW060229290526
45789CB00003B/1469